Amene FKI
Mounira HAJJAJI
Kaouthar JMAL

Psychosocial factors at work

Amene FKI
Mounira HAJJAJI
Kaouthar JMAL

Psychosocial factors at work

The contribution of the effort/reward imbalance model

This book is a translation from the original published under ISBN 978-620-6-71257-2.

Publisher:
Sciencia Scripts
is a trademark of
Dodo Books Indian Ocean Ltd. and OmniScriptum S.R.L publishing group

120 High Road, East Finchley, London, N2 9ED, United Kingdom
Str. Armeneasca 28/1, office 1, Chisinau MD-2012, Republic of Moldova, Europe
Printed at: see last page
ISBN: 978-620-7-61886-6

TABLE OF CONTENTS

INTRODUCTION

Over the last few decades, the organisational conditions of production in the world of work have changed dramatically, with work becoming more intensive, the pace of work more demanding, more multi-skilled and more flexible. Physical hardship, far from disappearing, has been coupled with considerable mental hardship. These changes have led to the emergence of new forms of psychological suffering, including stress at work(1). Work-related stress occurs "when there is an imbalance between a person's perception of the constraints imposed on them by their environment and their own resources for coping with them"(2). It is currently a public health problem, not least because of its deleterious effects and its proven human, organisational and societal costs (3).

This new representation of health at work militates in favour of identifying aspects of work organisation that are more harmful overall than others. This identification involves the use of validated theoretical models, which identify certain psychosocial dimensions of the work environment for which there is empirical evidence of their pathogenic power for exposed workers. As well as reducing the complexity of the psychosocial reality of work to significant components in terms of health risks, these models also facilitate the development and implementation of workplace interventions. There are currently two models of psychosocial risk that are internationally recognised for their considerable contribution to the production of consistent scientific knowledge on the importance of the links between social and psychological phenomena at work and the development of a number of diseases. These are Karasek's 'demand-autonomy-work support' model(4) and Siegrist's 'effort-reward imbalance' model(5). The "effort/reward imbalance" model conceptualised by Siegrist (5) at the end of the 1980s is based on the observation that a work situation characterised by a combination of high effort and low recognition is accompanied by pathological emotional and physiological reactions. Low levels of recognition may be economic (inadequate pay), social (lack of esteem and respect) or organisational (job insecurity and poor promotion prospects). This model predicts that the lack of reciprocity between costs and gains can lead to emotional stress. Siegrist (5) distinguishes two main categories of effort: extrinsic and intrinsic. Extrinsic stress corresponds to the demands of the job, and includes time constraints, interruptions, responsibilities, working hours, etc. extra work, physical workload, increased demand. Intrinsic effort (or over-investment) reflects the attitudes and motivations associated with excessive commitment to work. The individual's involvement in his work will therefore be greater, and he will mobilise more resources, including, according to Niedhammer and Siegrist (6), in situations where the gains will be relatively low. Work on Siegrist's model (5) has often been the subject of studies in the medical field(7,8).In this context, we proposed to undertake a study in a water exploitation and distribution company where the activities are characterised by the presence of physical and mental demands in order to meet the following objectives:

- Assessing stress levels at work using the imbalance model effort/reward in a population of workers.

- Research the socio-demographic and professional determinants associated with an effort/reward imbalance.

METHODS

1 Type of study :

The present study is a descriptive and analytical cross-sectional survey that took place in a district of the Société Nationale d'Exploitation et de Distribution des Eaux (SONEDE) in Sfax and conducted over a period of 2 months (from 01 December 2017 to 31 January 2018).

2 Study population :

The population studied was made up of workers employed by SONEDE in Sfax. They were divided into two distinct occupational classes: execution (technical) and administration. These two classes corresponded to different salary ranges, levels of education or training and jobs. The executive group represented all of the company's active employees whose activities were mainly manual (mechanics, plumbers, electricians, storekeepers, technical staff, lift operators, multi-skilled workers, drivers, security staff). Sedentary workers are those whose activity is office-based (administrative agents, engineers, technicians, accountants).A list of staff by name, age, working hours and departments was obtained from the Human Resources Management Department. Before the start of the study, and during a personal interview, each subject was informed of the objectives of the survey, as well as their right to refuse to take part, without having to give any justification.

2.1 Inclusion criteria :

Our study included :

- Adults aged between 20 and 60 and free of any psychiatric pathology.

- Participants who have given their informed consent.

2.2 Exclusion criteria :

We have excluded :

- Known carriers of psychiatric pathologies.

- Subjects who did not give informed consent.

3 Data collection

Data were collected using a questionnaire comprising the following sections (Appendix 1):

3.1 Socio-demographic characteristics

The questionnaire enabled us to collect descriptive variables relating to the main socio-demographic characteristics, in particular age, sex, weight, height, level of education (primary, secondary or university), marital status (single, married, divorced or widowed), children/dependent parents, etc.

3.2 Professional characteristics

We collected the following data: workstation, nature of tasks, seniority, number of hours worked per week, standby duty, etc.

Standby duty refers to periods during which the employee, outside normal working hours, must be available to carry out work for the company.

3.3 Lifestyle habits

We asked employees about their smoking and drinking status, as well as about their practising a leisure physical activity (APL). Referring to the recommendations of the World Health Organisation (WHO), we considered any physical activity equivalent to 30 minutes of active walking per day.

3.4 Medical history

We recorded the pathological history of our study population, in particular chronic pathologies and musculoskeletal disorders.

3.5 Measuring stress at work

The model used to characterise stress factors at work is Siegrist's Effort/Reward Imbalance model in its validated French version, comprising 23 questions(9,10). Responses for each item range from 1 to 4. This model focuses on a negative trade-off between 'costs' and 'benefits' at work. It has 3 dimensions:

❖ **Effort (score ranging from 6 to 30) :**

Contains 5 items (time constraints, interruptions, responsibilities, overtime, increased constraints) plus 1 item on physical workload, relevant to the positions held.

❖ **Awards (scores ranging from 11 to 55) :**

Includes 11 items: remuneration (1 item), esteem (5 items), control over professional status (job security and career opportunities) (5 items).

❖ Over-investment (score ranging from 6 to 24) :

Contains 6 items: "inability to get away from work", "difficulty relaxing after work".

The over-investment score is then dichotomised at the upper tertile of the distribution in the study sample, i.e. a threshold of 18 in our sample:

- <18: no over-investment

- ≥18: presence of overinvestment

❖ Building the effort/reward ratio

Ratio= 11/6 x effort score / (66 - reward score)

A ratio > 1 defines employees exposed to an imbalance between effort and reward.

4 Statistical analysis:

The data collected was entered and processed using SPSS20 software.

4.1 Descriptive study

In the descriptive section, we listed all the characteristics of the population studied. Qualitative variables were presented in the form of proportions, and translated into figures or tables. Quantitative variables were expressed as averages and limits.

4.2 Analytical study

A univariate analytical study was carried out to look for a relationship between the presence of an effort/reward imbalance and sociodemographic, occupational and medical characteristics. Statistical analysis was carried out using the Chi 2 test or the Ficher exact test to determine the relationship between two qualitative variables. Student's t-test was used to compare the means of two independent samples. The significance level was set at 5% and the differences were deemed significant at $p<0.05$.

5 Bibliographic research

The bibliographical search was carried out using the following search engines:

"In this section, we'll take a look at some of the k e y words used in our research: stress, effort/reward imbalance, work, psychosocial risks.

6 Ethical considerations

Patient anonymity was respected. The study was conducted with strict respect for medical confidentiality and without any conflict of interest.

RESULTS

1 Socio-demographic characteristics of the population studied

Eighty-one employees took part in the survey, representing a participation rate of 77.14% (81/105).

1.1 Age

The average age of employees was 42.49 +/- 11.34 years, with extremes ranging from 22 to 59 years.

1.2 Gender

The majority of workers were male (87.7%) (Figure 1).

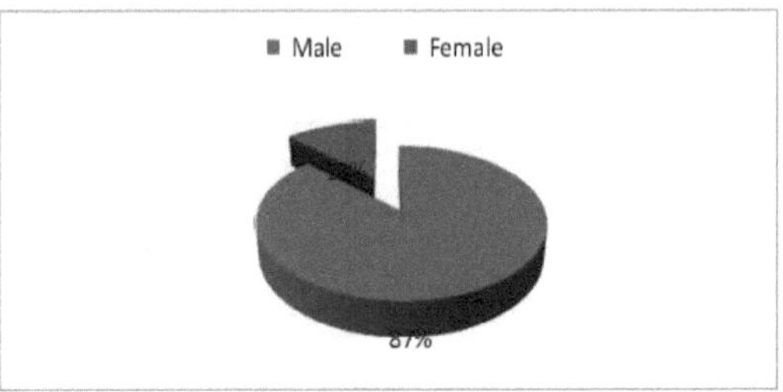

Figure 1: Breakdown of the study population by gender

1.3 Marital status

The majority of employees (76.5%) were married with a number of dependent children ranging from 0 to 4 and an average of 2.14 ± 1.62 children.

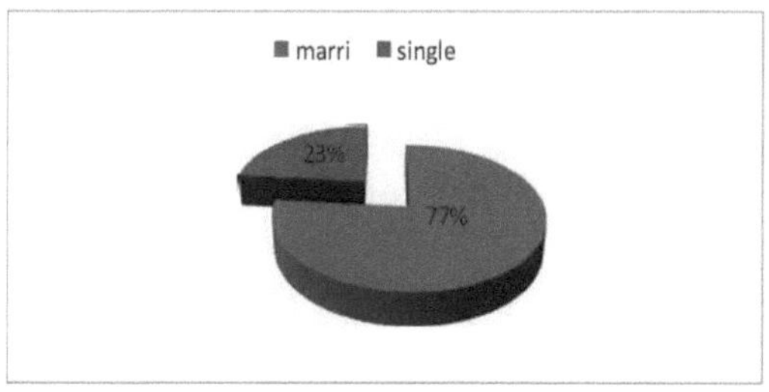

Figure 2: Breakdown of study population by marital status

1.4 Level of study

More than half the employees had secondary education (51.9%) (Table I).

Table I: Breakdown of the population by level of education

Level of study	Workforce	Percentage (%)
Primary	14	17,3
Secondary	42	51,9
University	25	30,9
Total	81	100

1.5 Distribution of the population by body mass index :

The average body mass index (BMI) was 24.68 ± 4.53 kg/m^2 with extremes of 17.43 and 40.25 kg/m^2 . Among the workers, 48.9% were overweight (BMI>25 kg/m^2) (Figure 3).

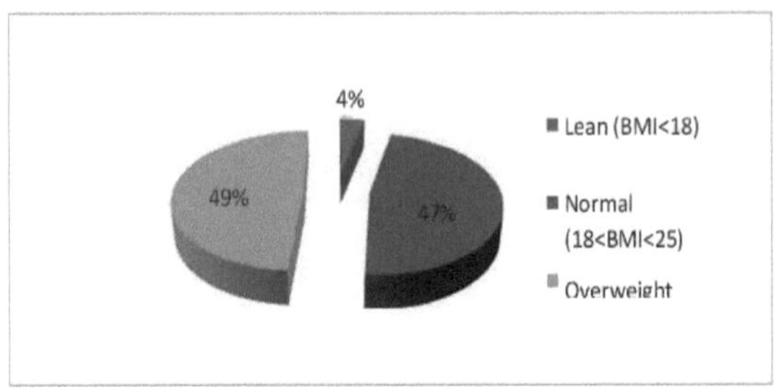

Figure 3: Distribution of workers according to BMI

2 Lifestyle habits

There were 44 smokers (i.e. 54.3% of employees), all of them male, with an average consumption of 22.5 cigarettes. Smoking was more common among active workers than sedentary workers (70.7% versus 37.5%), with a significant difference (p=0.003). The majority of employees (94.4%) drank coffee, with an average of 2 cups a day. Ten employees (12.7%) reported drinking alcohol. Of the 81 subjects included, 24 workers performed moderate LPA on a regular basis ($\geq$ 3 times a week, such as walking, cycling, gardening, etc.) and 18 subjects performed sustained LPA (football, weight training, etc.) at least once a week (Table II).

Table II: Distribution of the population according to physical activity level

	Workforce	Percentage (%)
No physical activity	39	48,1
Moderate physical activity	24	29,7
Sustained physical activity	18	22,2
Total	81	100

3 Professional characteristics :

3.1 Type of activity

The split between active and sedentary workers was almost equal (Figure 4).

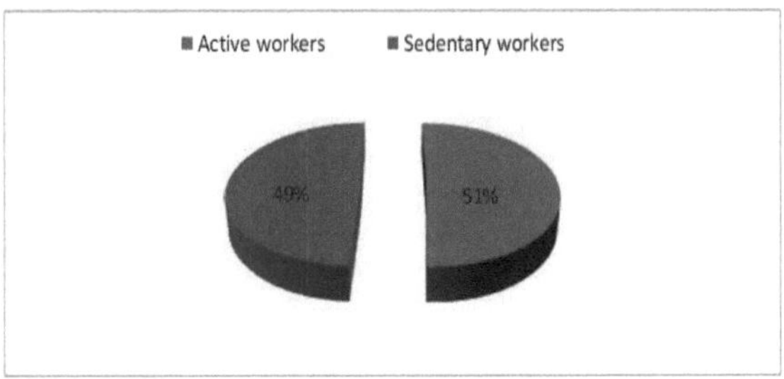

Figure 4: Breakdown of employees by type of activity

3.2 Workstation

The majority of sedentary employees were administrative staff (20.9%) and engineers (13.5%). The majority of active employees were mechanics (11.1%) and multi-skilled workers (7.4%) (Table III).

Table III: Breakdown of workers by workstation

Profession	Workforce	Percentage
Administrative agents	17	20,9
Engineers	11	13,5
Workers Section heads	4	4,9
Sedentary Technicians	6	7,4
Accountants	3	3,7
Mechanics	9	11,1
Warehousemen	6	7,4
Lifters	6	7,4
Active workers Multi-skilled workers	6	7,4
Plumbers	5	6,1
Turners	2	2,4
Drivers	2	2,4
Electrician	1	1,2
Security agent	1	1,2
Total	81	100

3.3 Length of service and working hours

The average length of service was 17.02 ±11.85 years and ranged from 1 to 38 years. years. Seniority of more than 20 years was found in 44.4% of workers (Figure 5).

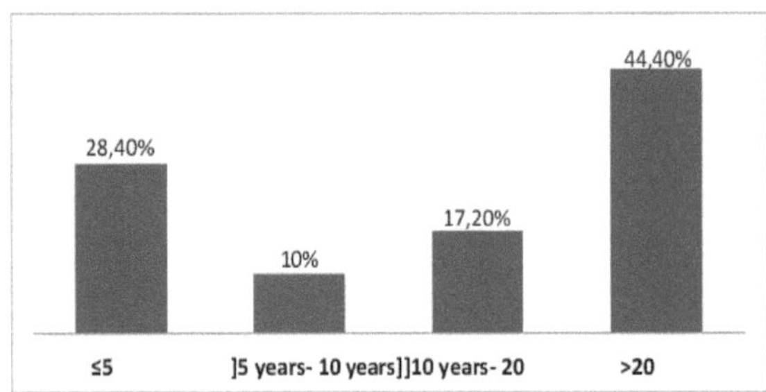

Figure 5: Breakdown of employees by length of service

The average number of hours worked per week was 40.84 ± 2.1 hours and varied between 40 and 50 hours/week. On-call duty concerned 17 employees (21%). Almost all employees (98.8%) took breaks during their work.

4 Medical history

A personal pathological history was reported by 37% of employees. These included chronic pathologies (hypertension, diabetes, dyslipidaemia) in 14.8% of cases and musculoskeletal disorders (MSD) in 9.8% of cases (Table IV).

Table IV: Breakdown of study population by medical history

History	Workforce	Percentage
HTA	8	9,9
Diabetes	2	2,5
Dyslipidemia	2	2,5
Asthma	4	4,9
Colon cancer	1	1,2
Thyroid cancer	1	1,2
Peptic Ulcer Disease	2	2,5
Lumbar hernia	5	6,1
Cervical hernia	1	1,2
Shoulder tendonitis	2	2,5

5 Evaluation of psychosocial constraints at work using the Siegrist model

5.1 Effort/reward imbalance

According to the Siegrist model, the average effort score was 15.35 ± 5.19 and ranged from 7 to 26, while the average reward score was 20.85 ± 8.12 and ranged from 8 to 44. An imbalance in the effort/reward balance (ratio > 1) affected 30.9% of respondents (Table V).

Table V: Distribution according to the presence or absence of an effort/reward imbalance Imbalance

effort/reward	Workforce	Percentage
Yes	25	30,9
No	56	69,1

5.2 Over-investment at work

The average over-investment score was 15.77 ± 3.25, with extremes of 7 and 23. Thus 30.9% of employees were over-invested in their work (score ≥ 18) (Table VI).

Table VI: Distribution according to the presence or absence of over-investment in work

Overinvestment	Workforce	Percentage
Yes	25	30,9
No	56	69,1

6 Risk factors associated with an effort/reward imbalance

The comparison between workers belonging to the high-risk group for effort/reward imbalance and those belonging to the low-risk group showed certain distinctive parameters between the two groups. These parameters were sex, BMI, level of education, type of activity, smoking, alcoholism and over-involvement in work. In fact, the group at high risk of effort/reward imbalance was male ($p=0.02$), had the highest BMI ($p=0.007$), no higher education ($p=0.024$), smoked ($p=0.002$), drank alcohol ($p=0.022$) and belonged to the group of active workers ($p=0.02$) (Table VII).

Table VII: Factors associated with an effort/reward imbalance

Effort/reward imbalance

No (n=56)		Number of employees (%)	Number of employees (%)	p	OR [95% CI]
			Yes (n=25)		
Age		41,48 ± 11,28	44,76 ± 11,28	0,23	-
Gender	Male	46 (64,8)	25 (35,2)	0,027	1,56 [1,31-1,85]
	female	10 (100)	0 (0)		
BMI		23,78 ± 3,56	26,98 ± 5,12	0,012	4,36 [1,57-11,42]
Situation	Single	15 (78,9)	4 (21,1)	0,29	-
matrimonial	Married	41 (66,1)	21 (33,9)		
Level of study	No	34 (60,7)	22 (39,2)	0,002	4,63 [1,85-14,22]
superior	Yes	22 (88)	3 (12)		
Smoking	No	32 (86,5)	5 (13,5)	0,002	5,33 [1,75-16,24]
	Yes	24 (54,5)	20 (45,5)		
Alcoholism	No	53 (73,6)	19 (26,4)	0,022	5,57 [1,26-24,54]
	Yes	3 (33,3)	6 (66,7)		
APL	No	22 (56,4)	17 (43,6)	0,31	-
	Yes	20 (47,6)	22 (52,4)		
Type of activity	Active	22 (53,7)	19 (46,3)	0,002	4,90 [1,69-14,08]
	Sedentary	34 (85)	6 (15)		
Seniority		16,80 ± 12,13	17,52 ± 11,42	0,80	-
On-call duty	No	47 (73,4)	17 (26,6)	0,10	-
	Yes	9 (52,9)	8 (47,1)		
Diseases	No	46 (70,8)	19 (29,2)	0,55	-
chronicles	Yes	10 (62,5)	6 (37,5)		
TMS	No	51 (68)	24 (32)	0,66	-
	Yes	5 (83,3)	1 (1,9)		

DISCUSSION

Occupational stress is now a genuine occupational health problem, encompassing a large number of symptoms and consequences. Since 1996, Siegrist's effort-reward imbalance model has enriched stress models by proposing an approach based on the dissonance between high costs and low gains. In this context, we conducted a descriptive and analytical study of employees in a district of the national water exploitation and distribution company in Sfax, the objectives of which were to describe the psychosocial constraints at work using Siegrist's effort-reward imbalance model and to identify the determinants associated with it.

1 Strengths and limitations of the study

The choice of the cross-sectional type of study stems from the need to recruit as many participants as possible, and has the advantage of being more practical because of its short duration and low cost. However, this type of study has a number of shortcomings. Indeed, the associations found may be a good source of etiological hypotheses without establishing a clear causal link. These results nevertheless reinforce those of other studies in the international epidemiological literature. We used the Siegrist questionnaire to detect any effort/reward imbalance in workers. This questionnaire, validated in French, identifies pathogenic working conditions as those combining high effort with low rewards.

The main advantages of this model over the Karasek model are that it takes personality factors into account and also looks at aspects of the individual's control over his or her career and job. However, given the educational level and poor command of French among some of the workers interviewed, we were unable to use this tool as much as a self-questionnaire, but the survey form was filled in by the interviewer, who tried as far as possible to maintain the same discourse and attitude with all the subjects. As in all studies, the information gathered by questionnaire is often subjective and reflects the worker's perception of his work experience.Finally, a bias in the composition of the sample cannot be completely ruled out. In fact, there is a selection bias due to some employees refusing to take part.

2 Socio-demographic and professional characteristics

The average age of the workers was 42.49 +/- 11.34 years. Subjects aged over 45 accounted for 50.6% of these workers. According to some authors, age is a determining factor in physical capacity at work. This decreases rapidly after the age of 45, making the perception of the efforts made increasingly arduous (11). The majority of employees (87.7%) were men. The low number of women is explained by the fact that this type of company employs more men, and this is dictated by the type of activity, which involves a large proportion of executive work. Women in this company work exclusively in office automation. This finding is similar to that found in the Samotrace survey, where men accounted for 86% of employees in the water, gas and electricity production and distribution sector(12). In terms of level of education, only 30.9% of the study population had a university degree. Mausner-Dorsh and Eaton concluded that the higher the level of education, the lower the psychosocial constraints (13).

Current smokers represented 54.3% of employees. This prevalence is comparable to that estimated by Fakhfakh R et al (14) among manual workers, service personnel, employees and middle managers (48.3% to 54.4%). However, it is much higher than that reported in a meta-analysis of 15 European studies involving 166,130 workers (smoking prevalence was 25%)(15). Smoking was more common among active workers than sedentary workers (70.7% vs. 37.5%; p=0.003). This result was consistent with several studies in the literature, such as a study of male Kôrin workers (16), in which the prevalence of smoking was higher in active workers than in office workers (OR= 2.00, 95% CI [1.43 -2.80]; RR= 1.33, 95% CI [1.12 -1.59]).On-call duty concerned 17 employees. A French study carried out at EDF-GDF had reported that the major constraint generated by on-call duty was telephone calls. These calls were five times more frequent during on-call weeks, resulting in shorter sleep (an average of 6.8 hours compared with 7.4 hours during normal weeks) and tiredness on waking (25.7% compared with 13.2%). Psychological balance and social and family life were also disrupted in the group of subjects who frequently worked on-call (linear and significant association) (17).

3 Psychosocial constraints at work

According to the European Agency for Safety and Health at Work, stress is the most widespread health problem in the world of work. Surveys conducted in the European Union provide alarming figures: 22% of employees suffer from stress at work. In his transactional model of the "imbalance between effort and reward", Siegrist (5) states that the best definition of chronic stress is to describe it as a disparity between the efforts made and the rewards obtained. Extrinsic effort is defined by Siegrist as work constraints such as time constraints, interruptions, responsibilities, physical load and increasing work demands. Intrinsic effort, or "over-commitment", corresponds to attitudes and motivations associated with an excessive commitment to work combined with a strong desire to be approved of and valued (5). As far as rewards are concerned, three dimensions of reward are important: monetary satisfaction, socio-emotional reward and control over professional status (i.e. promotion opportunities and job security).The prevalence of effort/reward imbalance in our study population was of 30.9%. In the literature, this prevalence varied according to the sector of activity (12). In a recent study, Keser et al(18) reported a prevalence of effort/reward imbalance of 45.8% among workers at a Turkish academic university. However, other authors have revealed much lower prevalences. Niedhammer's work in the gas and electricity production and distribution sector showed prevalences of exposure to effort/reward imbalance of 4.6 % in men and 5.8% in women (19). Similarly, the Samotrace survey (12) of 60056 employees in various sectors reported a prevalence of effort/reward imbalance of 2.8% in men and 3% in women. At national level, Kacem et al (20) revealed a prevalence of 16.7% in the telecommunications sector.The prevalence of over-investment at work in our study population was 30.9%. This result was consistent with several studies in the literature, such as the Samotrace survey (12), which reported a prevalence of exposure to over-investment of 33.7% in men and 38.9% in women, and the GAZEL(9) cohort, which revealed a prevalence of 36.18% in men and 41.18% in women.

4 Determinants of the effort/reward imbalance

4.1 Socio-demographic determinants

In our study, effort/reward imbalance was more frequent in men (p=0.027). This result was inconsistent with several studies which found that women were more frequently exposed to effort/reward imbalance. Indeed, Siegrist (21) revealed that work stress was more pronounced in women, particularly in the intrinsic component and the effort-reward ratio. Also, in a study conducted in Sweden (22), the effort/reward imbalance was more frequent among women working in the public sector. Similarly, in a Norwegian study, exposure to psychosocial factors was more frequent among women, which explains the higher rate of sick leave among these women(23).

The dominance of this imbalance among men in our study can be explained by the small number of women among the participants and the type of activity they engaged in (exclusively sedentary).

In our study, the group at highest risk of effort/reward imbalance had the highest BMI. Several studies had investigated the relationship between obesity and certain occupational factors such as work-related stress. According to Kouvonen et al (24), effort/reward imbalance was associated with a BMI ≥ 25 kg/m^2 (OR = 1.08, 95% CI: 1.02-1.15).

Stress can contribute to obesity through its effects on behaviour and metabolism. Authors have observed a significantly higher proportion of obese people among workers who have declared that they are subject to high levels of stress and strain at work (25). Previous research has shown that the onset of obesity can be directly linked to the biological effects of chronic stress, resulting in an accumulation of adipose tissue in the intra-abdominal region (26).

According to Park et al, obesity could also be caused by coping mechanisms that are harmful to health, such as overeating, physical inactivity and excessive alcohol consumption (27). High psychological workload may also be a causal factor in obesity, if it occurs in the absence of adequate social support at work. In addition, obese men were more likely than their normal-weight colleagues to report that their work required a lot of physical effort. This could explain the high prevalence of obesity among men in manual jobs (28). We also found that the effort/reward imbalance was associated with a low level of education (p=0.002). This result was consistent with the study by Niedhammer et al (9), who observed a relationship between effort and level of education among men, with effort increasing among the least educated. Rewards were also associated with level of education, with higher education graduates having the highest rewards for both men and women. A study of the ratio according to the same study also revealed that the prevalence of exposure to this imbalance was significantly lower among higher education graduates and managers.

4.2 Determinants linked to lifestyle habits

The effort/reward imbalance was more frequent in current smokers than in current non-smokers, with a statistically significant difference (p=0.002). This result was consistent with several studies reporting an association between effort/reward imbalance(29) and smoking. In a Finnish study of 46190 workers, Kouvonen et al (30) reported that a high effort/reward ratio was associated with smoking (OR= 1.28). After taking into account age, level of education, professional status, type of employment and marital status, employees who had more stress at work were found to be smokers more often than their colleagues who had less stress. Similarly, in a cohort study conducted in the United States, psychosocial stress was associated with smoking behaviour in working adults (31).However, other studies have not reported an association between work stress and smoking(32-35). Indeed, a study in India(36) did not reveal a significant association between the different domains of the effort/reward imbalance score and the presence of adductive habits.

In our study, alcoholism was also associated with effort/reward imbalance (p=0.026). According to some studies, alcoholism spares no socio-professional class. However, it is the most physically demanding professions: workers exposed to heat (forges, foundries, etc.), construction workers, farmers, warehouse workers, etc., and those in contact with the public: craftsmen, sales representatives and agents, postmen, police officers, etc., who are most likely to drink (37). Beyond individual predispositions, there are causes linked to the organisation and the people involved.working conditions that significantly increase the risk of alcohol abuse, such as a imbalance between effort and reward. In fact, all causes of stress are conducive to alcohol consumption, as alcohol has proven but transient anxiolytic properties. Work overload, too many responsibilities without the means to act, unrealistic deadlines and objectives are also among the constraints that encourage alcohol consumption (38).

4.3 Professional determinants

Active workers were more at risk of an effort/reward imbalance than sedentary workers (p= 0.02). This result is consistent with the GAZEL(9) cohort, which found that employees in the lowest occupational categories had the lowest rewards and the highest exposure to an imbalance between extrinsic effort and rewards (ratio of extrinsic effort to rewards > 1). These results were found for both men and women.

Some researchers have conducted their studies using samples of workers from several socio-economic levels in order to compare their degree of psychological distress. These authors placed manual workers at the lowest level on the hierarchical continuum. Other authors have studied blue-collar workers specifically under the heading of manual workers or unskilled workers (39).

Next, Caplan et al. compared the stress levels of four types of job, namely skilled blue-collar workers, unskilled blue-collar workers, white-collar professionals and white-collar non-professionals. The results showed that skilled blue-collar workers complained more of monotony and depression than the other groups studied. The authors attempted to explain this phenomenon by suggesting that these blue-collar workers were probably overqualified in relation to the requirements of their jobs. As a result, their skills could not be put to the test, leading to a perception of monotony, and the job was boring (40).

The aim of a study published by Wright et al was to look for correlations between environmental characteristics, psychological stress, satisfaction and symptoms of physical illness. The research was carried out among employees (n= 701 white-collar workers, n= 437 blue-collar workers) in Sweden. The results showed that blue-collar workers complained more of symptoms of physical and psychological illness, had the lowest levels of job satisfaction and suffered worse working conditions than white-collar workers. The authors concluded that poor working conditions increase dissatisfaction and stress levels, leading to the appearance of symptoms of physical and psychological illness (41). In fact, a prospective study published by Niedhammer and Siegrist (6) on 416 blue-collar workers, over a follow-up period of 6 and a half years, showed an association between effort/reward imbalance and an increase in the incidence of ischaemic heart disease. Similarly, in a cohort of 10,308 London civil servants followed over 5 years, the combination of The "high effort - low reward" approach was associated with an increased incidence of "high effort - low reward" disease. ischaemic heart disease (42). Several studies have estimated that between 10% and 40% of workers are exposed to some level of 'effort/recognition imbalance', mainly among employees from socio-economically disadvantaged groups (43). This lack of recognition undermines self-esteem and opens the door to psychological, physiological and behavioural manifestations, the mental health consequences of which can take the form of depression, burnout, high psychological distress or even suicide (44).

CONCLUSION

The theme of psychosocial factors at work in occupational risk epidemiology has grown considerably in recent years. The Effort/Reward Imbalance model has been developed to assess the psychosocial constraints of the work environment.

The water distribution sector is characterised by the presence of several occupational categories that correspond to different salary ranges, levels of education or training and jobs.

In this context, we conducted a survey of 81 workers, with the aim of describing the level of stress at work, based on the effort-reward imbalance model, and identifying the associated socio-demographic and occupational determinants.

Methodologically, we conducted a descriptive and analytical cross-sectional study among employees of a district of the national water exploitation and distribution company (SONEDE) in Sfax over a period of 2 months. Data were collected using a pre-established form containing socio-demographic characteristics, lifestyle habits, professional characteristics and medical history. The Siegrist questionnaire was used to assess psychosocial stress at work. The descriptive study was supplemented by an analytical study of the effort/reward ratio and the various demographic, occupational and medical parameters.

The average age of the workers was 42.49 +/- 11.34 years. The majority (87.7%) were male. Only 30.9% of employees had higher education. The average body mass index (BMI) was 24.68 ± 4.53 kg/m^2 , so 48.9% of the study population were overweight. Current smokers accounted for 54.3% of employees. Smoking was more common among active workers than sedentary workers (70.7% vs. 37.5%), with a significant difference (p=0.003).

Alcoholics accounted for 12.7% of the workers. Of the 81 subjects included, 51.9% of employees were engaged in leisure physical activity.

Active workers represented 51% of the study population and were mainly mechanics (11.1%) and multi-skilled workers (7.4%). Sedentary workers represented 49% of the study population and were mainly administrative staff (20.9%) and engineers (13.5%). The average length of service was 17.02 ± 11.85 years. All staff worked 40.84 ± 2.1 hours. On-call duty concerned 17 employees (21%). A personal pathological history was reported by 37% of employees. These included chronic conditions (hypertension, diabetes, dyslipidaemia) in 14.8% of cases and musculoskeletal disorders (MSDs) in 9.8% of cases.

Evaluation of psychosocial constraints at work using the Siegrist model revealed an average effort score of 15.35 ± 5.19 and an average reward score of 20.85 ± 8.12. An imbalance in the effort/reward balance (ratio > 1) affected 30.9% of respondents. In the literature, prevalence varied according to sector of activity. The average over-investment score was 15.77 ± 3, meaning that 30.9% of employees were over-invested in their work. This result was consistent with several studies in the literature, such as the Samotrace survey, which reported a prevalence of exposure to overinvestment of 33.7% in men and 38.9% in women. We investigated the factors associated with effort/reward imbalance in our study population. At the end of the analytical study, effort/reward imbalance was more frequent in male workers. This result was inconsistent with a number of studies that found that women were more frequently exposed to effort/reward imbalance. The dominance of this imbalance among men in our study can be explained by the small number of women among the participants and the exclusively sedentary type of activity they engaged in.

In our study, the group at highest risk of effort/reward imbalance had the highest body mass index. Several studies had found an association between obesity and certain occupational factors such as stress at work. We also found that the effort/reward imbalance was associated with a lower level of education (p=0.002). This result was consistent with some studies which have found that the prevalence of exposure to this imbalance was significantly lower among higher education graduates and managers.

Regarding the association of work stress with lifestyle habits, we found that effort/reward imbalance was more frequent in current smokers than in current non-smokers, with a statistically significant difference (p=0.002). This result was consistent with several studies reporting an association between effort/reward imbalance and smoking. In our study, alcoholism was also associated with effort/reward imbalance (p=0.026). This result was comparable to several recent bibliographical data which have approved that beyond individual predispositions, there are causes linked to the organisation and working conditions which significantly increase the risk of alcohol abuse, such as an imbalance between effort and reward.Active workers were more at risk of an effort/reward imbalance than sedentary workers (p= 0.02). Some authors have indicated that employees in the lowest occupational categories have the lowest rewards and the highest exposure to effort-reward imbalance. At the end of this study, we can conclude that the level of work-related stress linked to an effort/reward imbalance is high in this population.A comprehensive approach to prevention in the workplace aimed at reducing psychosocial stress is necessary. Furthermore, the success of interventions to reduce stress-related health problems in the workplace is difficult to dissociate from a more global public health policy. In particular, this policy should enable the establishment of a company surveillance system with the aim of identifying the extent of health problems linked to stress at work and being able to assess the effects of the improvement programmes implemented. This policy should also include legal and financial means to encourage companies to put in place appropriate preventive strategies to counter this pandemic affecting the Western world.

REFERENCES

1. Vezina M, Bourbonais R, Marchand A, Arcand R. Stress at work and mental health among Quebec adults. Canadian Community Health Survey; 2008. Available at http://www.stat.gouv.qc.ca/statistiques/sante/etat-sante/mentale/stress-travail.pdf

2. El Maalel O, Maoua M, Boughattas W, Zaouali M, Souissi A, Chatti S, et al. Study of work stress, salivary cortisol and cardiovascular risk in Tunisian bus drivers. Arch des Mal Prof l'Environnement. Elsevier Masson; 2011 Dec 1;72(6):623-32.

3. Hassard J, Teoh K, Cox T, Dewe P, Cosmar M. Calculating the cost of work-related stress and psychosocial risks. European Agency for Safety and Health at Work; 2014. Available on https://osha.europa.eu/en/tools-and-publications/publications/literature_reviews/calculating-the-cost-of-work-related-stress-and-psychosocial-risks

4. Robert K, Töres Th. Healthy Work: Stress, Productivity, and the Reconstruction of Working Life; 1990. Available at: https://www.questia.com/library/99885609/healthy-work-stress-productivity-and-the- reconstruction

5. Siegrist J. Adverse health effects of high-effort/low-reward conditions. J Occup Health Psychol. 1996 Jan;1(1):27-41.

6. Niedhammer I, Siegrist J. Psychosocial factors at work and cardiovascular

disease: the contribution of the Effort/Reward Imbalance model. Rev Epidemiol Sante Publique. Masson; 1998;46(5):398-410.

7. Bosma H, Peter R, Siegrist J, Marmot M. Two alternative job stress models and the risk of coronary heart disease. Am J Public Health. American Public Health Association; 1998 Jan;88(1):68-74.

8. Peter R, Geißler H, Siegrist J. Associations of effort-reward imbalance at work and reported symptoms in different groups of male and female public transport workers. Stress Med. John Wiley & Sons, Ltd; 1998 Jul 1;14(3):175-82.

9. Niedhammer I, Siegrist J, Landre MF, Goldberg M, Leclerc A. Étude des qualités psychométriques de la version française du modèle du Déséquilibre Efforts / Récompenses. Epidém. et Santé Publique. 2000; 48: 419-437

10. Siegrist J, Starke D, Chandola T, Godin I, Marmot M, Niedhammer I, et al. The measurement of effort-reward imbalance at work: European comparisons. Soc Sci Med. 2004 Apr;58(8):1483-99.

11. Kang D, Kim Y, Kim J, Hwang Y, Cho B, Hong T, et al. Effects of high occupational physical activity, aging, and exercise on heart rate variability among male workers. Ann Occup Environ Med. 2015 Dec 25;27(1):22.

12. Cohidon C, Arnaudo B, Murcia M, Centre DS. Malaise and psychosocial environment at work: initial results of the Samotrace programme, company section, France. Bull Epidemiol Hebd 2009;25- 26:265-9.

13. Mausner-Dorsch H, Eaton WW. Psychosocial work environment and

depression: epidemiologic assessment of the demand-control model. Am J Public Health. 2000 Nov;90(11):1765-70.

14. Fakhfakh R, Hsairi M, Achour N. Epidemiology and prevention of tobacco use in Tunisia: a review. Preventive Medicine. 2005; 40: 652- 657

15. Nyberg ST, Fransson EI, Alfredsson L, Bacquer D De, Bjorner JB, Hamer M, et al. Job Strain and Tobacco Smoking: An Individual- Participant Data Meta-Analysis of 166 130 Adults in 15 European Studies.PLoS ONE. 2012;7(7).

16. Kim BG, Pang DD, Park YJ, Lee JI, Kim HR, Myong JP, et al. Heavy smoking rate trends and related factors in Korean occupational groups: analysis of KNHANES 2007- 2012 data. BMJ Open. 2015;5(11):e008229.

17. Imbernon E, Warret G, Roitg C, Chastang JF, Goldberg M. Effects on health and social well-being of on-call shifts. An epidemiologic in the French National Electricity and Gas Supply Company. J Occup Med. 1993 Nov;35(11):1131-7.

18. Keser A, Li J, Siegrist J. Examining Effort-Reward Imbalance and Depressive Symptoms Among Turkish University Workers. Work Heal Saf. 2018;XX(X):1-6.

19. Niedhammer I, Chastang J-F, David S, Barouhiel L, Barrandon G. Psychosocial Work Environment and Mental Health: Job-strain and Effort-Reward Imbalance Models in a Context of Major Organizational Changes. Int J Occup Environ Health. 2006 Apr 19;12(2):111-9.

20. Kacem I, El Maalel O, Maoua M, Boughattas W, Omrane A, Ben Amor I, et

al. Evaluation of Mental load of teleoperators in a Tunisian call center. Ann Med Psychol (Paris). 2018;

21. Siegrist J, Wahrendorf M, Goldberg M, Zins M, Hoven H. Is effort-reward imbalance at work associated with different domains of health functioning? Baseline results from the French constances study. Int Arch Occup Environ Health. Springer Berlin Heidelberg; 2018;

22. Social S, Agency I, Unit SA, Institutet K. Effort - eward imbalance , overcommitment and their associations with all-cause and mental disorder long-term sick leave - a case- control study of the swedish working population. Int J Occup Med Environ Health. 2016;29(6):973-89.

23. Sterud T. Work-related gender differences in physician-certified sick leave: a prospective study of the general working population in Norway. Scand J Work Environ Health. 2014 Jul;40(4):361-9.

24. Kouvonen A, Kivimäki M, Virtanen M, Heponiemi T, Elovainio M, Pentti J, et al. Effort-reward imbalance at work and the co-occurrence of lifestyle risk factors: Cross- sectional survey in a sample of 36,127 public sector employees. BMC Public Health. 2006;6:1-11.

25. Brunner EJ, Chandola T, Marmot MG. Prospective effect of job strain on general and central obesity in the Whitehall II Study. Am J Epidemiol. 2007 Apr 1;165(7):828-37.

26. Schulte PA, Wagner GR, Ostry A, Blanciforti LA, Cutlip RG, Krajnak KM, et al. Work, obesity, and occupational safety and health. Am J Public Health.

2007 Mar;97(3):428-36.

27. Park J. Work stress and performance. Stat Canada. 2007; 5-19

28. Park J. Obesity and work: Stat Canada. 2009; disponible sur:

https://www150.statcan.gc.ca/n1/pub/75-001-x/2009102/article/10789-fra.htm.

29. Peter R. . Job stressors, coping characteristics, and the development of

coronary heart disease (CHD): results from two studies.

PsychologischeBeitrage. 1995;37:40-5.

30. Kouvonen A, Kivima M, Virtanen M, Pentti J, Vahtera J. Work stress,

smoking status, and smoking intensity: an observational study of 46 190

employees.J Epidemiol Community Health. 2005; 59(1): 63-9.

31. Slopen N, Zobel Kontos E, Ryff CD, Ayanian JZ, Albert MA, Williams DR.

Psychosocial stress and cigarette smoking persistence, cessation, and relapse

over 9-10 years: A prospective study of middle-aged adults in the United States

NIH Public Access. Cancer Causes Control. 2013;24(10):1849-63.

32. Landsbergis PA, Schnall PL, Deitz DK, Warren K, Pickering TG, Schwartz

JE. Job strain and health behaviors: results of a prospective study. Am J Health

Promot. 1998 Mar 26;12(4):237-45.

33. Reed DM, LaCroix AZ, Karasek RA, Miller D, MacLean CA. Occupational

strain and the incidence of coronary heart disease. Am J Epidemiol. 1989

Mar;129(3):495-502.

34. van Loon AJ, Tijhuis M, Surtees PG, Ormel J. Lifestyle risk factors for

cancer: the relationship with psychosocial work environment. Int J Epidemiol.

2000Oct;29(5):785- 92.

35. Netterstrøm B, Kristensen TS, Damsgaard MT, Olsen O, Sjøl A. Job strain and cardiovascular risk factors: a cross sectional study of employed Danish men and women. Br J Ind Med. 1991 Oct;48(10):684-9.

36. Priyanka R, Rao A, Rajesh G, Shenoy R. Work-Associated Stress and Nicotine Dependence among Law Enforcement Personnel in Mangalore , India. Europe PMC. 2016;17:829-33.

37. Carrie N. Relevance in occupational medicine of screening questionnaires used to assess risky or harmful alcohol consumption . 2015.

38. Darshan M, Raman R, Ram D, Annigeri B, Sathyanarayana Rao T. A study on professional stress, depression and alcohol use among Indian IT professionals. Indian J Psychiatry. 2013 Jan;55(1):63.

39. Cadieux V. Les facteurs professionnels entraînant de la détresse psychologique chez les cols bleus. Mémoire numérisé par la Direction des bibliothèques de l'Université de Montréal.2005;

40. Caplan RD, Cobb S, French Jr JRP, Harrison R Van. Job demands and worker health: Main effects and occupational differences. Washington: U.S. Department of Health, Education and Welfare; 1975 (U.S.G.P.O. Stock No. 1733-00083).

41. Wright I, Bengtsson C, Frankenberg K. Aspects of psychological work environment and health among male and female white-collar and blue-collar workers in a big Swedish industry. J Organ Behav. John Wiley & Sons, Ltd;

1994 Mar 1;15(2):177-83.

42. Siegrist J. Risques psychosociaux : outils d ' évaluation de lasituation de travail perçue. Références en santé au Travail. 2015;142:109-12.

43. Siegrist J. Reducing social inequalities in health: work-related strategies. Scand J Public Health. SAGE PublicationsSage UK: London, England; 2002 Sep 25;30(59_suppl):49-53.

44. Stansfeld S, Bosma H, Hemmingway H MM. Work characteristics predict psychiatric disorders: prospective results from the Whitehall II Study. Occ Env Med. 1999;56:302- 7.

APPENDICES

Survey form

1- Socio-demographic characteristics

Age years

Sex: male □ female □

Weight kg **height** :m **BMI** kg/m2

Marital status: single□ Married□ Divorced □ Widowed□

Dependent children: no□ yes□

Level of education: Primary □ Secondary□ University□

2- Lifestyle habits :

Smoking: no□ yes□ Age of onset years

Still smoking□ Has stopped smoking □

Smoking history: years. Number of cigarettes/day: Quantity PA

Alcohol: no □ yes□ Quantity:

Coffee: no□ yes□ number of coffees/day:

Do you regularly (≥3 times a week) engage in physical activity or sport?

No □ yes□

3- Professional features

Position:

Length of serviceyears

Type of work: manual activity □ office activity □

Working hours: morning□ afternoon□ night□

Number of hours worked per week:

Breaks during work: no□ yes□

Standby duty: no□ yes□

4- Medical history :

High blood pressure □ Diabetes □dyslipidemia □musculoskeletal disorders□

Other antecedents:

French version of the Effort-Reward Imbalance questionnaire - 2004

For any use, please quote these two references:

Niedhammer I, Siegrist J, Landre MF, Goldberg M, Leclerc A. Etude des

qualités psychométriques de la version française du modèle du Déséquilibre

Efforts/Récompenses. Revue d'Epidémiologie et de Santé Publique

2000;48:419-437

Siegrist J, Starke D, Chandola T, Godin I, Marmot M, Niedhammer I, Peter R.

The measurement of effort-reward imbalance at work: European comparisons.

Social Science and Medicine 2004;58:1483-1499

1I'm constantly pressed for time because of a heavy workload

Disagree倭1 Agree, and I'm not disturbed at all. 倭2

Okay, and I'm a little confused 倭3

Okay, and I'm confused 倭4

Okay, and I'm very confused 倭5

2I am frequently interrupted and disturbed in the course of my work

Disagree倭1 Agree, and I'm not disturbed at all. 倭2

Okay, and I'm a little confused 倭3

Okay, and I'm confused 倭4

Okay, and I'm very confused 倭5

3 I have a lot of responsibility at work

No agreement 倭1

Right, and I'm not at all perturbed 倭2

Okay, and I'm a little confused 倭3

Okay, and I'm confused 倭4

Okay, and I'm very confused 倭5

4 I'm often forced to work overtime

Disagree倭1 Agree, and I'm not disturbed at all. 倭2

Okay, and I'm a little confused 倭3

Okay, and I'm confused 倭4

Okay, and I'm very confused 倭5

5 My job requires physical effort

No agreement 倭1

Okay, and I'm not confused at all................................倭2

Okay, and I'm a little confused 倭3

Okay, and I'm confused 倭4

Okay, and I'm very confused 倭5

6 Over the last few years, my work has become increasingly demanding.

Disagree倭1 Agree, and I'm not disturbed at all. 倭2

Okay, and I'm a little confused 倭3

Okay, and I'm confused 倭4

Okay, and I'm very confused 倭5

7 I get the respect I deserve from my superiors

Agreed...倭1

Disagree, and I'm not at all disturbed 倭2

Disagree, and I'm a little disturbed 倭3

I disagree, and I'm disturbed 倭4

I don't agree, and I'm very disturbed 倭5

8 I get the respect I deserve from my colleagues

Agreed 倭1

Disagree, and I'm not at all disturbed 倭2

Disagree, and I'm a little disturbed 倭3

I disagree, and I'm disturbed 倭4

I don't agree, and I'm very disturbed 倭5

9 At work, I receive satisfactory support in difficult situations

Agreed 倭1

Disagree, and I'm not at all disturbed 倭2

Disagree, and I'm a little disturbed 倭3

I disagree, and I'm disturbed 倭4

I don't agree, and I'm very disturbed 倭5

10 I'm treated unfairly at work

No agreement 倭1

Right, and I'm not at all perturbed 倭2

Okay, and I'm a little confused 倭3

Okay, and I'm confused 倭4

Okay, and I'm very confused 倭5

11I am experiencing or expecting an undesirable change in my life.

work situation

No agreement 倭1

Okay, and I'm not confused at all................................倭2

Okay, and I'm a little confused 倭3

Okay, and I'm confused 倭4

Okay, and I'm very confused 倭5

12 My prospects of promotion are poor

No agreement 倭1

Right, and I'm not at all perturbed 倭2

Okay, and I'm a little confused 倭3

Okay, and I'm confused 倭4

Okay, and I'm very confused 倭5

13 My job security is under threat

No agreement 倭1

Right, and I'm not at all perturbed 倭2

Okay, and I'm a little confused 倭3

Okay, and I'm confused 倭4

Okay, and I'm very confused 倭5

14 My current job corresponds well to my training

Agreed..倭1

Disagree, and I'm not at all disturbed 倭2

Disagree, and I'm a little disturbed 倭3

I disagree, and I'm disturbed 倭4

I don't agree, and I'm very disturbed 倭5

15 Given all my efforts, I receive the respect and esteem I deserve for my work

Agreed..倭1

Disagree, and I'm not at all disturbed 倭2

Disagree, and I'm a little disturbed 倭3

I disagree, and I'm disturbed 倭4

I don't agree, and I'm very disturbed 倭5

16 Given all my efforts, my prospects for promotion are good.

Agreed	倭1
I don't agree, and I'm not at all perturbed...	倭2
I disagree, and I'm a bit confused	倭3
I disagree, and I'm disturbed	倭4
I disagree, and I'm very disturbed	倭5
17 Given all my efforts, my salary is satisfactory Agreed	倭1
I don't agree, and I'm not at all perturbed...	倭2
I disagree, and I'm a bit confused	倭3
I disagree, and I'm disturbed	倭4
I disagree, and I'm very disturbed	倭5

18 At work, I often find myself

I totally disagree

No agreement

Agreed

Absolutely

Agreed

pressed for time............................倭1倭2倭3倭4

19 I'm starting to think about problems at work as soon as I get up in the

morning............倭1倭2倭3倭4

20 When I get h o m e , it's easy for me to relax and forget about my work.

everything about my job..............倭1倭2倭3倭4

21 Those close to me say I sacrifice too much

for my work...................................倭1倭2倭3倭4

22Work is still on my mind

when I go to bed.................................倭1倭2倭3倭4

23When I put something off that I should be doing on t h e day, I have a

hard time. trouble sleeping at night..............................倭1倭2倭3倭4

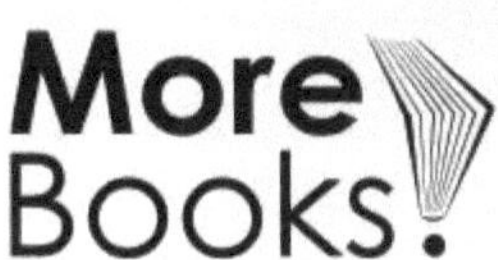

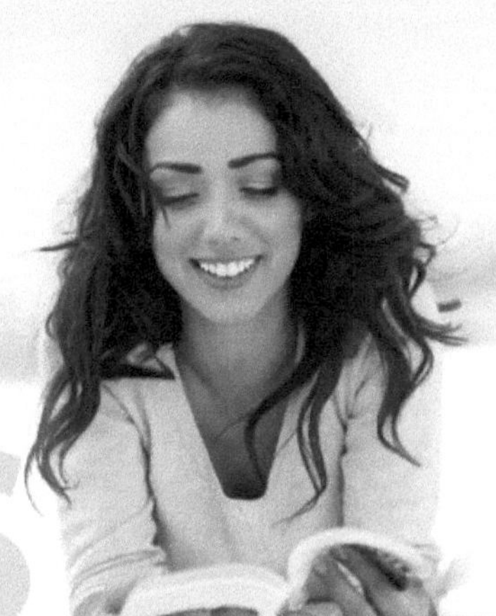

yes
I want morebooks!

Buy your books fast and straightforward online - at one of world's fastest growing online book stores! Environmentally sound due to Print-on-Demand technologies.

Buy your books online at
www.morebooks.shop

Kaufen Sie Ihre Bücher schnell und unkompliziert online – auf einer der am schnellsten wachsenden Buchhandelsplattformen weltweit! Dank Print-On-Demand umwelt- und ressourcenschonend produziert.

Bücher schneller online kaufen
www.morebooks.shop

info@omniscriptum.com
www.omniscriptum.com

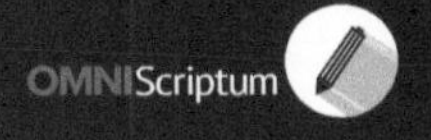

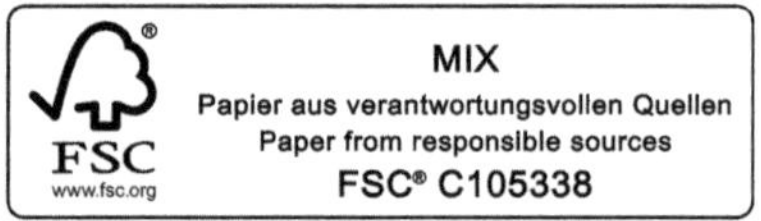

Printed by Books on Demand GmbH, Norderstedt / Germany